MW00892380

Radiant Health

6 Easy Things You Can Do to Achieve and Keep It

What, Why and How

By Jane Bersie

Radiant Health

Introduction

You can achieve and maintain radiant health. You don't have to be a 'perfect' person to do so, and you don't have to spend all of your time working at it. In this book I discuss six important areas of habits that have worked for me to boost my health, feelings of wellness, energy levels and positive outlook. These are not fads that come and go; they are solid proven methods based on evidence and extensive scientific research recommended by reputable authorities. Even if you choose to only adopt some of these suggestions, your general wellness can be improved with each area incorporated.

Change often can be difficult, especially when one is attempting to change very ingrained habits. So what makes these things 'easy' as described in the subtitle of this book? Change gets easier if you are shown what to change, are shown compelling evidence for the change, and are shown how to incorporate the change into your life. When you see the great benefits that can be achieved by making incremental changes in your behavior, change becomes easier.

This publication is intended to broaden your understanding of health and wellness and help you make informed choices of health options. It is not intended as a replacement for medical treatment or therapy by any physician or licensed health care provider. Always consult your physician or qualified health-care professional on matters regarding your

Radiant Health

personal health before adopting any suggestions in this book.

Congratulations *on purchasing this book and investing in your health! As a thank-you gift, go to http://www.radiance4u.com/ for a calming music mp3 download with affirmations to relax and reinforce the healthy behaviors discussed in this book. Please do not listen to this music while driving or when your full attention is necessary for an activity. To get your free mp3 download now go to http://www.radiance4u.com/*

Table of Contents

Introduction iii

Table of Contents v

Chapter 1: Exercise 1

Chapter 2: Sleep 6

Chapter 3: Nutrition 12

Chapter 4: Mind and Body 21

Chapter 5: Breathing 29

Chapter 6: Attitude 36

Chapter 7: Conclusion 40

Chapter 1: Exercise

"I decided to take an aerobics class. I bent… twisted… gyrated… jumped up and down… and perspired for a half an hour. But by the time I got my tights on…. the class was over!" - Anonymous[1]

In order to be healthy, you have to move your body. We weren't designed for continuous inactivity. Your physical body is a marvelously complex piece of machinery/energy/chemistry that can adapt itself to whatever you ask of it. Research has shown that if you continually stress one side of your body, without stressing the other side, bone gets stronger on the stressed side, and bone gets eaten away by enzymes on the non-stressed side. This happens because what is not needed is a waste of body resources to keep. The old 'use it or lose it' adage applies here. You don't have to be a super jock or a fitness nut to be healthy; you just have to incorporate physical activity into your life. And, if you do not, your health will suffer.

According to the Centers for Disease Control and Prevention adults need a **minimum** of 2.5 hours (150 minutes) of moderate exercise or 1.5 hours (90 minutes) of intense exercise, plus 2 hours of strength training each week to maintain health. Currently only 20% of American adults meet these guidelines.[2] Double the minimum times to gain even more health benefits.

Radiant Health

"Regular physical activity is one of the most important things you can do for your health. It can help:

- Control your weight
- Reduce your risk of cardiovascular disease
- Reduce your risk for type 2 diabetes and metabolic syndrome
- Reduce your risk of some cancers
- Strengthen your bones and muscles
- Improve your mental health and mood
- Improve your ability to do daily activities and prevent falls, if you are an older adult
- Increase your chances of living longer"[3]

Regular exercise has been likened to 'the fountain of youth'. When you exercise at least moderately:

- Your heart rate goes up, giving your heart muscles a workout making them stronger, allowing it to pump more blood per beat so it doesn't have to work as hard all the time.
- Circulation increases by having the muscles push the venal blood back to the lungs and heart.
- Breathing increases, saturating your blood with more oxygen to feed every cell in your body.
- Toxins are more easily eliminated from each cell due to the increased circulation.
- All your muscles and bones and connective tissue get stronger from use.
- Your lymph system works better by squeezing the lymph back to the lymph nodes. The lymph

nodes filter and clean the lymph and produce more T-cells to boost your overall immunity.
- Your brain produces endorphins to make you feel better.
- You sleep better because you give your physical body a chance to get tired.
- You burn more calories moving your muscles, which helps you lose weight, or lets you eat more.
- All your systems start working better to give you more energy for everything else.

So how do you get started? Start slow, don't overdo it or you will get sore and achy and stop before it becomes a habit. Keep it simple. Go for a walk -- ten minutes at a time works. Sneak it in any chance you get. If you work in an office building, climb steps up one floor or down two instead of taking the elevator. If you are elderly in the cold weather, try to get to an indoor mall to do your walking. If you love music, take a dance class, or just turn on some music and dance in your house.

There are many community sponsored classes for physical fitness. Try gentle yoga. You don't have to turn yourself into a pretzel to do yoga. If you like yoga, you can work your way into more intense classes as you go along. Yoga has the added benefit of incorporating the strengthening requirement into the workout. You use your body working against gravity to strengthen your muscles. For any physical fitness class, if you don't like the teacher, try a different one until you find somebody you like that makes you want to go back. Classes can be fun and give you a chance to socialize too. The

Radiant Health

advantage of taking a class is that they are harder to skip than totally relying on exercising on your own.

If you can't get to a class, there are free online exercise videos to follow or videos to purchase. Public TV has exercise programs to follow along with too. Gardening, for example, is good exercise -- if you have the opportunity and like to do it. The main point is that once you get started, the more you incorporate exercise (movement) into your life, the easier it gets and the more you will want to continue to do it because you will just feel better.

Last year I injured my knee and had knee surgery. I hobbled around pretty much all summer. Since I really couldn't exercise with my legs, I went kayaking. Using my upper body for paddling, my heart rate went up and I still got my exercising in, including the strength training of pushing the paddle through the water. If you want to badly enough, you can find a way to exercise. If you can find an exercise buddy, it's even better. Anything that helps you to exercise regularly will increase the likelihood that you will incorporate it into your life.

For one week, keep track of how much time you are moderately or vigorously making an effort to move your body (at least 10 minutes at a time) spread over at least four days per week. Use this to determine if you are deficient. You can also use it to develop a strategy to get more exercise if you need it. See what you can honestly trade out of your life (an extra ½ hour of TV or internet a day for example) to make time for exercising

– both cardio and strength. If you don't make it a priority, it's not going to happen. **Make the commitment now.**

Chapter 2: Sleep

"Get at least eight hours of beauty sleep — nine if you're ugly."- Betty White[4]

The general recommendation for adults is 7-8 hours of sleep per night, and according to the National Institutes of Health, 1/3 of all American adults get less than that. If you think that missing 1-2 hours of sleep per night won't affect you, other than being a little tired, think again.

"Sleep plays a vital role in good health and well-being throughout your life. Getting enough quality sleep at the right times can help protect your mental health, physical health, quality of life, and safety. The way you feel while you're awake depends in part on what happens while you're sleeping. During sleep, your body is working to support healthy brain function and maintain your physical health. ... The damage from sleep deficiency can occur in an instant (such as a car crash), or it can harm you over time. For example, ongoing sleep deficiency can raise your risk for some chronic health problems. It also can affect how well you think, react, work, learn, and get along with others."[5]

Because during sleep your body is repairing your heart and blood vessels, sleep deficiency can raise your risk for heart problems, high blood pressure, kidney disease, diabetes and stroke. By interfering with the regulation of your hungry/full hormones, sleep deficiency increases you risk of obesity. By interfering with your insulin uptake, sleep deficiency results in higher blood sugar, increasing your risk of diabetes.

"Sleep also supports healthy growth and development … [releasing] a hormone that promotes normal growth … [it] boosts muscle mass and helps repair cells and tissues. Your immune system gets compromised when you don't get enough sleep. Studies have shown that sleep deficient individuals have more trouble fighting common infections."[6]

Quality sleep prepares your brain for learning and remembering by forming new neural pathways each night. It also can affect how well you solve problems, make decisions, pay attention, be creative, control your emotions and behavior, cope with change, and are motivated. Don't compromise your quality of life and health by compromising your quantity and quality of sleep.

So maybe you want to sleep better and longer, but either you can't fall asleep when you want to, or you wake up in the middle of the night, or you wake up early and can't get back to sleep. Here are some tried and true tips for improving the quality of your sleep, to maximize your sleep benefits.

Tips for getting better quality sleep.

- Go to bed at the same time every night as much as possible. This trains your internal clock and circadian rhythms. Get up at the same time too.

- Get some exercise and sunshine during the day to get better sleep at night. "Researchers in Northwestern University's Department of Neurobiology and Physiology reported that adults who exercised aerobically four times a week improved their sleep quality from poor to good."[7] [8] Do not, however, exercise vigorously just prior to sleeping as you may have trouble winding down enough to rest.

- Be careful about eating close to bedtime as sugar, caffeine (coffee, chocolate, tea, sodas) and a too-full stomach can interfere with your sleep. The effects of caffeine can last as long as 8 hours. Indigestion from too spicy or rich foods can interfere with your sleep too.

- Develop rituals prior to sleep that can quiet your mind and prepare your body for sleep. Examples would be quiet reading, meditation, listening to calming music, taking a calming (not too hot) bath, drinking herbal tea, or practicing deep breathing. All of these rituals work to calm your nervous system.

- "Avoid watching TV or using your computer in the evening, at least an hour or so before going to bed. These devices emit blue light, which tricks your brain into thinking it's still daytime".[9] Also, the content may be too stimulating to prepare yourself for sleep. Your subconscious continues to be affected by these images even after you have gone to sleep.

- Keep your bedroom environment quiet, dark, cool and comfy. For sleeping, the National Sleep Foundation (NSF) recommends that "Your bedroom should be cool – between 60 and 67 degrees."[10] You want your body core to cool down for sleep, so adjust the temperature, your blankets and sleepwear with this goal in mind.

- A white-noise machine, calming music, or even ear plugs can help block unwelcome sleep-disturbing noises.

- Use blackout drapes to keep your bedroom as dark as possible. Turn off, remove or at least cover up all the blinky, buzzy electronic gadgets in your bedroom. "Even the slightest amount of light in the white or blue bandwidths is enough to seriously depress your pineal gland's production of melatonin for the night, which is why sleeping in total darkness is so important. Melatonin is important for the proper functioning of your immune system, scavenging free radicals, reducing inflammation, and helping your body to rid itself of cancer cells; multiple studies point to the role of melatonin in protecting you from multiple types of cancer, including breast cancer."[11] If you have to get up at night, use a dim red-colored night light because it won't interfere with your melatonin production, and you will have an easier time getting back to sleep.

- Finally, adjust your mattress, pillows and bed linens to provide you with the coziest and comfiest sleeping environment possible for you. "Kids and dogs are the biggest bed hogs and some of the worst sleepers. Both deserve their own sleeping space—and you deserve yours."[12] [13]

De-stress before sleeping. Nothing helps a good night sleep better than peace of mind. If you resolve what is bothering you before you go to bed, the 'chitta vritti' or mind chatter won't go round and round and keep you from falling asleep. Meditation helps to stop the mind chatter. Turning your problems over to a higher power, appreciating your problems as opportunities for growth, and just letting go, all contribute to the calmness that allows you to fall asleep. Remind yourself that your current situation will still be there when you awaken, and nothing can be accomplished by worrying and losing precious sleep.

If you are a night worker, or even worse, are required to alter your shifts, it takes about two weeks to reset your body clock to a new schedule. If possible try to remain on one shift consistently. If you change shifts every two weeks, you will always be off cycle. If you work a night shift, try to recreate a normal day/night schedule with room darkeners while you are sleeping and sunshine and exercise when you are not. You should be able to, with trial and error, figure out what works best for your health and sleeping ability. I use a Verilux (full spectrum) lamp for reading. It provides me with a little 'sunshine' even in the depths of winter.

Chapter 3: Nutrition

"Never eat more than you can lift." – Miss Piggy[14]

What to eat is a loaded subject. There are more 'diets' these days than you can count, with as many contradictions as there are 'diets'. Chocolate is good for you, oh no, chocolate is not good for you. Eggs are bad, oh no, now eggs are good. Finally people just think, "Scr#w it, I'm going to eat whatever I want." Instead of doing that, here are some healthy-eating guidelines. Ultimately you will still eat whatever you want, but it's good to consider what you are eating before you put it in your mouth.

I am not a nutritionist, but I have been eating and staying healthy for a good many years. I weigh about the same (or a little less) than I did in high school, about 50 years ago and, so far (fingers crossed), I do not have to take medications for health issues. Follow these guidelines most of the time. It is what you do over and over that affects your health the most, not the occasional slipup or splurge. It is also better to eat and drink a wide variety of foods. That way if something is good for you, you will get the benefit, and if something is bad for you, you won't get so much of it.

Be nice to yourself and your body, it's the only one you have. And remember there is no such thing as 'free'. If it is fat free, there is something being put in the food to make it taste and feel like fat, and that something is probably not as good for you as the original natural fat or oil was. Sugar-free has the same problem. Look, if you want to eat something, eat the real thing and be honest with yourself about how many calories it has. Don't try to fool yourself. When it comes to eating, honesty is the best policy. Oh yes, what on earth is non-fat cream? Milk with some thickeners – I guess. Here are my recommendations:

Water: Drink lots of clean water and eat foods high in water such as fruits and vegetables. Your body is made of up to 60% water. You lose it through sweating, breathing, and elimination. Water is essential for all your bodily functions to work. Mild to moderate dehydration is likely to cause thirst, tiredness, dry skin, headache, constipation, and light-headedness. We sometimes mistake thirst for hunger. The best way to tell if you are drinking enough water is to look at your urine. If it is clear you are probably hydrated, if it is very yellow, you need to start drinking more water. And don't wait until you are thirsty, because you are already dehydrated if you are thirsty.

I personally like to drink filtered water. I have a filter in my refrigerator. I try to keep my water in a non-leaching container with me most of the time. I don't like plastic bottles because I'm always leaving them around where they get hot and then the water tastes funny to me. The bottles are awful for the environment and totally unnecessary. Next time you drive by a dump, with huge piles of refuse being pushed around by bulldozers, think about eliminating plastic water bottles from your life, what a waste! Oh, and I like my water filtered because my body needs the water, but not all the other stuff that seems to come along with ordinary tap water these days. One more note about water, the film of tears (water) over your eyes is part of the lens of your eye. When you are dehydrated, this film dries out too, and you can't see as well. Have you ever noticed when you got emotional and 'teared' up a little, you could suddenly see more clearly. You can see more clearly all of the time if you stay hydrated.

Synthetic Chemicals: If it's chemical and man-made, try not to ingest it. I asked my doctor about drinking diet soda when I was pregnant. She said, "We know what sugar does to the body, it's been around a long time, it just makes you fat. The artificial stuff however, we just don't know what it does really". Actually I don't drink much soda at all. It's one of those cheat things. I might have one once every two months or so, and then I think, "Why did I drink that?" Our ancestors got us to now by eating plants and animals – i.e. natural stuff. Why start messing around with a million years of evolution? Read the labels. If it looks like a chemical cocktail, move along.

Although, the other day I was fooled by some bread. I like my bread to have very little ingredients so I usually put back the product when the ingredient list looks too long, but this time I read what was in it. Everything looked like nutritious food and was recognizable so I bought it. I have another pet peeve when it comes to food: dyes. According to the Center for Science in the Public Interest: "Commonly used food dyes, such as Yellow 5, Red 40, and six others, are made from petroleum and pose a 'rainbow of risks'. Those risks include hyperactivity in children, cancer (in animal studies), and allergic reactions."[15] I just don't want to be eating petroleum products.

Unprocessed Food: Try to eat fresh unprocessed food. Simple is better. Think about it. What do you think is better for you, an apple (minimal processing here) or applesauce that has been skinned, sliced, diced, mashed, heated until every bit of whatever was good in it is cooked away, flavored, colored, preserved for long shelf life and packaged in plastic or a can that could eventually leach into the food? Ok, I'm oversimplifying and I'm sure the applesauce people are trying to keep their product as nutritious as possible (with a really long shelf life), but you get the point. One good bit of advice is to shop around the outside isles of the supermarket because that is where all the fresh food is found. The inside isles are usually processed, packaged, preserved and dead.

Variety: Eat a variety of food. Another 'foody' piece of advice is to try to eat a 'rainbow of colors every day'. And by 'rainbow', I'm not talking about the dyes mentioned in the previous bullet points. For example, I'll pick a red pepper, an orange orange, a yellow banana, a green something or other and some blueberries to put in my cart. Natural brightly colored food is chock full of anti-oxidants and is good for you. Fresh turmeric stains everything it touches bright orange, maybe that's why it has such great anti-inflammatory properties. One more comment about 'processed' foods. White flour is processed to the point they take out all the nutritious part (the wheat kernel). White sugar is processed too. If the color is supposed to be the good stuff, where did the color go? Processed out I guess.

Greens: Eat your vegetables – mostly the green ones. They are probably the very best things you can be eating period. I am not a vegetarian, but most of what I eat is vegetables, legumes, some high quality grains and nuts and some fruit. I still have fish, chicken and meat, but not every day and when I do it's a small portion. I eat dairy and eggs too. If you want to lose weight in a healthy way (not too fast and not too crazy by only eating one type of food), chow down on lots of different kinds of vegetables. You can eat at least 1/3 bushel of broccoli for about the same amount of calories in a large bacon cheeseburger, large fries and large soda. The broccoli is better for you. You will feel full and not need to eat again for a long time – but please don't eat a 1/3 bushel! To me, most of a hamburger is the pasty white-flour bun. The fries are greasy and salty. Try eating a fry after it is cold, you'll see what I mean. The soda is a mostly high-calorie sugared or artificially-sweetened fizzy water. You have to drink a lot of water to flush a soda out of your system.

Oils: Keep your oils and fats un-hydrogenated. Even unprocessed coconut oil has been found to be better than partially-hydrogenated or hydrogenated oils. Remember when coconut oil was getting such a bad rap? They found out it was the processing that made it bad for you, and now it is back on the 'good for you' list – but only if it is non-processed. I like olive and flax oil too.

Fast food and polyunsaturated vegetable oils: safflower, corn, sunflower, sesame, cottonseed, peanut and soybean oils contain a lot of omega-6 fatty acids and contain little or no omega-3 fatty acids. Before the advent of fast food and the availability of plant oils, Americans consumed about equal amounts of omega-6s and omega-3s. Now, "Most American diets provide more than 20 times as much omega-6 [as] omega-3 fatty acids. There is general agreement that individuals should consume more omega-3 and less omega-6 fatty acids to promote good health."[16] According to Dr. Andrew Weil "This dietary imbalance may explain the rise of such diseases as asthma, coronary heart disease, many forms of cancer, autoimmunity and neurodegenerative diseases."[17] To get a better ratio, cut down on fast and processed foods, use olive oil instead of the high omega-6 oils listed here, and eat more fatty fish and omega-3 eggs.

Prepare your own: Cook – but not too much 'frying'. I just took a cooking class. The chef told us that restaurants, unless they are really good ones, tend to buy and serve the least expensive ingredients, increasing their profit margin and staying in business. Thus the food is probably not as high in quality as what you would cook for yourself at home. Once you get used to real fresh-food cooking (instead of just heating up some processed stuff) you will eat better for less and you will know what's in it.

In keeping with the philosophy of eating as many different kinds of foods as possible, here is a list of suggested foods to include in your diet. After listing them, I'm amazed at how many different kinds of good food are available, and I've only included fairly common foods eaten in the United States.

Spices and herbs: For example: basil, thyme, oregano, rosemary, turmeric, ginger, sage, clove, cinnamon, chili peppers, saffron, horseradish, fennel and lemongrass. Spices have naturally occurring chemicals that aid digestion, are anti-inflammatory, and have a host of other properties that are generally good for you. Plus they taste good and add 'spice' to your food and life.

Green food: Celery, cilantro, parsley, zucchini, cucumber, all kinds of lettuce, spinach, Chinese greens, bok choy, chards, broccoli, kale, brussel sprouts, cabbage, green peppers, okra, green beans, green peas, snap peas, olives, sprouts, lentils, pumpkins seeds, chlorella, seaweed (nori , wakame), and teas (tulsi, green, and peppermint). My grocery store carries a lot of different kinds of Asian greens that I am always afraid to buy because I don't know how to cook them (like bittermelon). Guess what, I should be a little more adventurous and learn. Oh yes, eat the other colored veggies too.

Fruits and berries: Apples, bananas, blueberries, cherries, raspberries, blackberries, strawberries, grapes (and raisins), apricots, peaches, pears, plums, kiwi, pineapple, papaya, mango, pomegranates, cantaloupe, oranges, lemons, limes, figs, dates, watermelon, tangerines, cranberries and avocados.

Mushrooms: button, crimini, enoki, shiitake, oyster, portabella, reishi, maitake, morels, truffles, and chanterelles. Mushrooms contain powerful compounds (beta-glucans) which help activate and modulate your immune system.

Beans and Legumes: adzuki beans, black beans, black-eyed peas, fava beans, butter beans, calico beans, chickpeas (garbanzo beans), edamame (soy beans), great northern beans, Italian beans, kidney beans, lentils (red, yellow, and green), lima beans, mung beans, navy beans, pinto beans, soy beans, split peas and peanuts.

Nuts, grains and seeds: Nuts: pistachios, walnuts, hazelnuts, Brazil nuts, pecans, almonds, macadamias, cashews, coconuts and pine nuts. Grains: Barley, oats, rice (brown or wild), wheat (whole), triticale, millet, amaranth, quinoa, and popcorn. Seeds: flax, chia, sesame, sunflower and buckwheat.

Fermented foods: Yogurt, kefir, sauerkraut, kimchi, kombucha, miso, tempeh, pickled vegetables: cucumbers, beets, radishes, and corn relish; wine, beer and sourdough bread. Check that the 'pickled' foods are really fermented and have not just had vinegar added. These foods usually contain active probiotics, which are good for your gut, and consequently your immune system. Note: Keep the wine and beer in moderation please.

A final confession: Yes, I try to eat the good stuff. I don't always. I like ice-cream and eat a little almost every day. I also keep some small dark chocolates in my freezer for occasional treats. Even a little coffee everyday is supposed to be good for you. In general, my choices usually include nutritious, unprocessed, fresh organic (when possible) food. It tastes good and makes me feel good, and that is what I normally like to eat. When I do indulge, it is in moderation. It is not hard to eat well; you just have to make a habit of **choosing** to eat better. Remember it's what you do every day that matters, not the occasional splurge.

Chapter 4: Mind and Body

"You should sit in meditation for 20 minutes a day, unless you're too busy, then you should sit for an hour" - Old Zen saying

If you think of your body as a just a complex physical/chemical mechanism, which by the way is pretty much how scientists and the medical profession look at it; then it's somewhat like a car or a computer. If you start to hear a clunk when you are driving, you take your car in, have it diagnosed, get it fixed by replacement or repair, and you merrily go along your way until you take it for another 'checkup' i.e. oil change and diagnostics if something else goes wrong. We too tend to think about the body like this. If your computer goes on the blink, it could need a software update, it could have contracted a virus, or maybe it needs a new part. Once again you fix it to continue to use it, or you get a new one -- which is not yet an option if our body goes completely out of whack. Nowhere in this mechanical/chemical model do you get anything close to the concept of a mind-body connection.

But the mind-body connection is another major component to health that is just as important as exercising, sleeping, and eating well. Your thoughts affect your body and your body affects your thoughts. Think for a minute. You are watching a scary movie and something happens on the screen that is building up to a scare, or scares you. Your heart starts to pound, your breath becomes more shallow, your stomach tightens with anticipation, your blood pressure rises and you might even start to clench your jaw because of the on-screen tension. There's no real threat happening. No monster is going to jump out of the closet to 'get' you. Watching the movie, your mind is creating all those physical changes happening in your body.

People used to say about some illnesses, "Oh it's just psychosomatic." Meaning, "They are not really sick; it's all in their head." Well, just because it starts in your mind doesn't mean there are not actual physical bodily results manifested. This is exactly what we are talking about as part of the mind-body connection. Here is a little experiment you can try, to see how the body can affect the mind. Breath is one of the most powerful mind-body connectors we have. Long slow deep diaphragmatic breathing calms the nervous system. Short fast shallow breathing causes anxiousness and excites the 'fight or flight' response in the nervous system.

Start out by taking a minute or two of slow deep breaths. When you inhale, your lower abdomen expands out, then your rib cage expands all around, and finally your collar bones lift up at the end. On an exhale, you gently push all the air out of your lungs (draw your stomach in too) and carefully get the last little bit of air out at the end (but don't force it). You will probably feel more relaxed than when you started. Now try a minute or less of fast very shallow breathing, panting and only allowing the air to come into the top part of your lungs. You will most likely become uncomfortable and mentally agitated. When we are upset, we tend to exhibit fast shallow breathing, but which comes first?

The reason I had you do this exercise is to show you that the 'mind-body' connection is real, not new-age woo-woo stuff. Thoughts and emotions affect your physical body and vice-versa. And if you want to optimize all aspects of your health, you will need to pay attention to your thoughts and emotions too. Dr. Mario Martinez, a Clinical Psychologist who practices in the field of psycho-immunology cites studies that show that watching acts of violence (on TV or the movies) suppresses our immune system (in terms of lower amounts of anti-bodies in the blood) for several hours. But, he has also found that people with a positive outlook on life recover their anti-bodies faster than negative-outlook (cynical) people do. On the other hand, according to Dr. Martinez, watching comedies or acts of kindness boosts the immune system. "Real laughter is contagious, comes from the belly, and is extremely healthy for you."[18] You might consider what your daily dose of the evening news is doing to you. Negative emotions and negative thinking depress your immune system. Positive feelings give your immune system a boost. Stress makes your blood ph more acidic, laughing makes it more alkaline. Alkaline blood helps you stay healthy.

If you want to feel happy, put a smile on your face. It stimulates your brain into feeling happier. Once again, which comes first, and does it really matter? I remember in one of his seminars, Tony Robbins gave an example of a woman who came to him for help, telling him she was very depressed. He noticed that her posture was extremely slumped over. He told her to put her shoulders back and stand up straight because it is almost impossible to feel depressed when you are standing up straight like that.[19] Try it yourself, put your head down, round your shoulders and slump down. Your breathing becomes shallower. You will start to feel more depressed. I always thought I was just the wrong height for airplane seats because the head-rest made me slump over, but now I think it's more of a deliberate method for keeping passengers docile (at least the short ones).

In Chinese medicine, certain emotions are associated with specific organs in the body. The theory is that emotions affect the immune, nervous and endocrine systems, which in turn create chemicals in the body that affect specific organs. A person who is constantly angry will tend to have liver problems because the liver has to work harder to get rid of the 'anger' created chemicals. People who live in fear tend to have kidney problems. Emotional stress promotes stomach and digestive problems. "He couldn't stomach that." Depression affects the lungs and respiratory system. When you are disappointed in love, it's popularly called 'a broken heart' and you have a higher tendency for heart problems.

Also over-excited emotions affect the heart too. Master Chunyi Lin of Spring Forest Qigong[20] says "Don't give your 95 year-old grandfather a surprise birthday party." Studies have shown that there is a higher correlation between people who hate their jobs and heart attacks than any other indicators – such as high cholesterol, etc. Most heart attacks occur on Monday morning when people are faced with having to go back to work to a stressful job they dislike.

Dr. Martinez also explains how our thoughts send signals to the immune system and that our immunity depends upon our beliefs. "The immune system is a confirmer of the consciousness you project. A defenseless consciousness creates a defenseless immune system. If you tell yourself, 'I don't want to feel anger anymore' i.e. repressing and controlling an emotion instead of experiencing and getting rid of it, your immune system will pump endorphins into your blood, keeping them high on a chronic basis to keep you from feeling. High endorphins in your blood affect your glucose metabolism; your glucose goes up; your insulin goes down and you have a much better chance of developing type 2 diabetes."[21] And we all thought it was just our genes and our diet.

Dr. Carolyn Myss, in her seminar on energetic healing[22], explains the mind-body connection in a different way. She gives an analogy: Every day you start out with a finite amount of energy, like a hundred dollars. You can spend that energy any way you choose i.e. living, getting your work and projects done, socializing, etc. But if the energy (thoughts and emotions) is being spent on old hurts, old resentments, and issues from the past that haven't been resolved, or the energy is being spent on worrying and fear for the future, then there is very little energy left to live right now, today. In fact, she says, you can go into an energy deficit, using up the energy your body needs to stay healthy, which eventually can result in an illness.

Both Dr. Myss and Dr. Martinez suggest that you should examine your health issues to try to see what benefit you get from having them. For example: if you have a cold, you don't have to go to work or school that day. There's no 'blaming' here, we all do this to a certain extent. You didn't consciously catch that cold, but maybe deep down, there was something at school or work you were avoiding, or you felt you were working too hard, and catching a cold allowed you a break to rest. You should also look at what the illness is keeping you from doing. If you are afraid, then the illness fulfills its purpose by allowing you to not do the thing that you didn't want to do. So much of our behavior is 'unconscious', and yet, when we dig deep enough into ourselves, the light bulb of awareness can turn on.

I'm **not** saying that all illness are **only** caused by emotional factors, but it is worth examining our thinking processes and emotions in order to understand all of the aspects of our health so we can stay healthier.

So, how do we cultivate positive emotions and get rid of negative emotions to try to keep our immune systems running well? The number one way to deal with your emotions in a positive (non-repressive) way is to first notice that you are having an emotion. Dr. Martinez says, "See how it feels in your body and just breathe into the tension you feel."[23]. Once you do that for a while, the tension lessens, and you can let it go. This is not necessarily easy, but can be learned just like anything else with practice.

This method works on past issues too. If you allow yourself to feel the hurt in your body that you felt when you were first hurt (shamed, betrayed or abandoned) , continue to feel it, breathe into it, plus try to see what good came from it, you will be able to let it go. Once you let it go, the physical manifestation of the issue usually resolves itself too. Dr. John E. Sarno in his book *Healing Back Pain*[24] discusses how stress, anxiety and repressed anger can sometimes be the cause of chronic pain and he explains mind-body methods to facilitate healing.

Another way to put a positive spin on your experiences is to cultivate a mindset that allows you to take a larger view. Master Chunyi Lin of Spring Forest Qigong says that the key to health and healing is love, kindness, and forgiveness.[25] Dr. Martinez tells us to cultivate the 'Four Immeasurables', which are: Loving Kindness -- toward yourself as well as others, Empathic Joy – celebrating the successes of others without jealousy or envy, Compassion -- wanting other people (as well as you) to end their suffering, and Equanimity – (the middle way) i.e. balance, this also includes balancing your giving to others against what you yourself need.[26]

Radiant Health

In *The Seven Spiritual Laws of Success*, Deepak Chopra counsels us to practice acceptance. "Today I will accept people, situations, circumstances, and events as they occur. I will know that this moment is as it should be because the whole universe is as it should be. I accept things as they are this moment, not as I wish they were. I take Responsibility for my situation and for all those events I see as problems. I know that taking responsibility means not blaming anyone or anything for my situation (and this includes myself). I also know that every problem is an opportunity in disguise, and this alertness to opportunities allows me to take this moment and transform it into a greater benefit." [27]

Cultivate an awareness of what is here and now. Cultivate an attitude of acceptance of what is here and now. And finally, cultivate an attitude of gratefulness for what is here and now. Your body will thank you for it.

Chapter 5: Breathing

"Unless it's your last breath, make it a good one."–
Jane Bersie

What is so important about breathing that it gets a whole chapter by itself in this book? After all, we automatically breathe about 20 thousand times a day. And when I say 'automatically' I mean it. This function is so important to staying alive that, just like your heart beating, your body takes care of it without any conscious thought on your part. If you quit breathing for about four minutes your brain is dead, another two minutes and you are dead.

The whole purpose of breathing is to get oxygen, which makes up about 20% of the air, into your lung's alveoli. The alveoli are the tiny sac-like end-points of your lungs that interface with blood vessels to get the oxygen hooked up with the red blood cells. If you could spread out your alveoli, they would cover a football field. "Ninety percent of metabolic oxygen comes from breathing. Ten percent comes from food."[28] Once in the blood stream, the oxygen gets delivered to each of the 37.2 trillion cells in your body.[29] We are talking national debt kind of numbers here. In case you forgot, a trillion is a million million, so there are 37 million million cells that need the oxygen you breathe.

Not every cell in your body needs oxygen -- your hair, nails, and the outermost layer of your skin are already dead and don't need it anymore, but the rest of them do, especially your brain and heart muscles. "This oxygen uptake by the cells is so important to survival that breathing a hydrogen cyanide concentration of 2000 parts per million will kill a human in about 1 minute. The toxicity is caused by the cyanide ion, which halts cellular respiration."[30] Another side note here is that cigarette smoke contains cyanide and smokers have about 2.5 times more cyanide in their blood than non-smokers. In addition, the toxins from smoking gunk up the alveoli too, which also decreases the oxygen amounts that can get to the blood and then to the cells.

Besides supplying critical oxygen to your cells, breathing also expels the carbon dioxide waste product produced by cell metabolism. Insufficient removal of carbon dioxide causes it to be taken up by the blood instead of the oxygen. This creates acidic blood, acidic cells, central nervous system damage, permanent deterioration of respiratory functions, and eventually death. So proper exhaling is just as important and inhaling. In fact, in some of the breathing classes I have taken they say that you can't get a good inhale, unless you've cleared the way first by a good exhale.

Now the wonderful thing about breathing is that besides being controlled automatically, it can also be consciously controlled. It's probably the only critical body function that works this way. Unlike the gurus who study in a cave for 10 or 20 years to control their heartbeat, you can learn to be a better breather in just a few hours or days. Adopting a habit of breathing better not only is easy to learn and costs you nothing --

so far the air is free. Once you learn better breathing, you can turn it back over to the 'automatic' side, and only notice you are not doing it when your consciousness interferes – like when you are stressed or upset. "If you learn to breathe effectively, you will improve the quality of your entire life."[31]

So, what constitutes 'better breathing'? First of all, breathe through your nose. "Western medical researchers have found a variety of benefits that come from breathing through the nostrils rather than the mouth. First, breathing through the nostrils results in more oxygen being absorbed into the arteries. This occurs because nitric oxide is made by our nose and sinus membranes and carried into our lungs during nostril breathing. Nitric oxide relaxes and widens the arteries, enabling them to absorb more oxygen. This gas, when inhaled even in small amounts into the lungs, can increase oxygen absorption significantly."[32] Breathing through your nose also results in cleaner, warmer, and moister air coming in to your body. "In a miracle of heat-efficiency, the air reaches body temperature within a little more than an inch of the outside world, even on a cold day."[33] You miss all that pre-treatment, breathing through your mouth.

When you breathe through your nose, your nose hairs catch and filter pollutants. The mucous membranes and cilia lining all the passageways trap pollutants. The white blood cells in the mucus hunt and kill off microbes, and the cilia (waves of fine hairs in the mucous) work against gravity to move the debris back up, dumping it off to the stomach for removal. The moisture from your out-breath is trapped in the mucus, and gets picked up by the next in-breath. The out-breath gets rid of the excess carbon-dioxide, the exhaust from cellular respiration, which can poison your system if not completely exhaled.

Less than a tenth of a liter of blood flows through the top of the lungs every minute, compared with 2/3 of a liter per minute in the middle. But down at the bottom of the lungs, well over a liter flows through each minute. "If you can learn to breath even a little bit better, you will notice immediate, profound shifts in your physical, mental, and emotional well-being."[34] So, how do you get the oxygen down to the part of the lungs that interacts with most of the blood? You do it by diaphragmatic breathing. If you watch a baby breathe, the baby's stomach rises while breathing in, and goes back down when breathing out. For some reason everybody starts out breathing this way, then by the time we reach high school, unless we have had some training, most of us become shallow breathers, i.e. keeping the stomach in while trying to breathe from only the top part of the chest. This adds tension to the body, robs us of a lot of needed oxygen, and keeps us from fully expelling the toxins and carbon dioxide.

I went to a Catholic grade school. We had choir almost every day, we learned to breathe deeply when we were singing. I think the nuns were onto something. Most yoga classes are also a good source of learning how to breathe properly. The science of yogic breathing is called 'pranayama'. It is one of the best things about taking a yoga class. This is how I teach breathing in my yoga classes. When you do this exercise, the only way you can do it wrong is if you are trying too hard, so just do this gently, slowly, and easily. Don't jerk and don't do it too strenuously.

Lie down on the floor on your back with your knees bent and your feet flat on the floor -- about hip width apart. Having your knees bent eases the pressure on your back. Rest your hands on the floor and relax your belly, i.e. just let it hang out. Close your eyes for a moment and get comfortable in this position. If you have to move around a bit go ahead to get the most comfortable you can be. You can do this in bed too if getting down on the floor is too hard for you, but it is easier to feel the movement on the floor.

Cow: Try gently to arch your back so there is a little space between your mid-lower back and the floor. In yoga this is called cow position. It might help to stick your belly out a bit. What you are doing is rocking your pelvis. Notice that in this position, the lowest part of your tailbone is touching the ground. If you were standing, your butt would be sticking out. Then go back to neutral position.

Cat: Next try to flatten your lower back against the floor. What you are doing is rounding your entire back, rolling the tailbone so the bottom part of it comes up and the mid-lower back is on the floor. You are tucking your tailbone. Pull your stomach in a little too. This yoga move is called cat because it resembles a cat when it rounds its back and hisses. Then go back to neutral position.

Once you have practiced cow and cat so you feel comfortable doing them, gently and smoothly alternate them so the transition starts to come naturally and easily. If you are having trouble doing this on the floor, you can get on your hands and knees, hands under shoulders, and try the cat/cow first this way to get the hang of it. Then try it with your back on the floor again.

Now, put your hands on your lower belly, and slowly take a deep breath so you see your hands raise up, and your belly sticking out. See how far you can get it to expand without straining. Next, slowly exhale so your belly naturally drops back down. At the bottom of the exhale you can pull your belly in just a little to get a little more air out, but once again **don't strain** and don't hold your breath when your lungs are full, or when your lungs are emptied. Practice this until you feel comfortable. If you get a little dizzy or tired, or you are trying too hard, just rest for a bit and breathe normally before trying again.

Finally, with your hands on your lower belly, breathe in slowly (through your nose) and watch your hands go up, expanding your belly out, where the air has to go, while also doing cow (arching your back a little) at the same time. Then expand your whole rib cage out (all around) and finally grab a little more air with your collarbones. When you breathe out slowly (through your nose), let your collarbones relax, let your ribs release, and let your belly go in (watch your hands go down) while doing cat (round your back a little) to help push out the air. Once again **don't strain**.

Note: to get up off the floor roll over to one side and rest in a fetal position until your body equalizes a bit, then with your top hand, push yourself up to sitting.

That is essentially belly or diaphragmatic breathing. When you feel sufficiently comfortable with it on the floor you can try to do the same thing sitting in a chair, and then standing up. If you get dizzy, quit for a while until the feeling goes away. Belly breathing feels a little different upright than lying on the floor because gravity isn't helping quite as much on the exhale, but your body should remember the moves. Easy does it, the cow/cat movements will be hardly noticeable when you are doing it correctly in an upright position.

There is only one other thing to remember about belly breathing. It takes a while for your body to do this automatically. You do have to practice. When you first start practicing regularly, you will easily slip back into your old habits, and you must remind yourself to consciously do it. Once it becomes second nature, the only time you have to remember to breathe this way is when you are stressed or upset and you slip back into shallow breathing. Just remembering to breathe this way and taking a few deep breaths will ease tension in your body. You might also notice feeling better, looking better and having more energy. It just makes sense when you are getting more oxygen to your 37.2 trillion cells with your in-breath and getting rid of more waste with your out-breath.

Chapter 6: Attitude

"You'll never find a rainbow if you are looking down."[35] – Charlie Chaplin

Exercising has been shown to release endorphins in the body, which trigger positive feelings. When you consider how you feel without a good night's sleep, you can safely say that: a good night's sleep improves your outlook on life and makes you happier. Proper nutrition positively affects your brain and mood. Think about how irritable you can get when you are hungry, or have been eating lots of junk-food. We are definitely happier when our body is pain free and healthy. And finally, the breathing experiments described in this book give you a direct experience of how good posture and diaphragmatic breathing make you feel better.

All of the things suggested in this book work synergistically to improve your positivity and your health; and a positive outlook on life has been shown to improve your health. According to the Mayo Clinic: a positive attitude and optimism on the state of your health may help you live longer with less depression, less stress, increased immunity to the common cold, better cardiovascular health, more coping skills and increased physical well-being.[36]

I recently visited my Aunt who was about to celebrate her 100th birthday. She was still living at home alone, although her daughter was right next door to help out. I fondly remember Barbara over the years as being a very gracious cheerful lady. We had a pleasant two-hour chat over lunch. I asked her what her secret was for living a long, relatively healthful life. She told me that, even though she had survived three heart attacks and was having some difficulty walking and was currently using a cane, she said that she just didn't let things bother her. And, she added, that she was also stubborn. I noticed, too, that she relied a great deal on her religious faith and thrived on her relationships, particularly with her children and grandchildren. Granted, even though she is only one person, and not a scientific study, 100 years of experience, in my opinion, is valuable.

I want to touch on the points she brought up. 'Not letting things bother you' certainly fits in with the idea that less stress is conducive to health, happiness and longevity. Psychologists tell us that it is not the external events of your life that cause stress, but your response to them. An example would be a school bell. If you were unfamiliar with a school bell ringing, the loud noise would startle you. But, when the school bell is perceived as a non-threatening normal event, you don't have that reaction. Another example would be a traffic jam. Your response to the jam determines your stress level. You have a choice to get angry and frustrated at the traffic jam, or, since you can't really do anything about it, you can just relax (by breathing deeply) and just go with the flow. This takes practice, but now you have the awareness and breathing skills to manage your responses.

Radiant Health

When my Aunt said that she was stubborn, I was reminded of a lecture I attended in the 70's by Professor John P. Brantner on how to live a long life. He said that a stubborn, idiosyncratic personality was necessary because it took a certain amount of determination and tenacity to keep on living, overcoming life's obstacles. Even though we tend to think of 'stubborn' as a negative trait when it shows up in others, stubborn really means a person who has a strong sense of self – and a lot of life-force. We build up our life force by achieving and maintaining our health.

You don't have to have 'religious faith' to be healthy, but having a belief in things outside yourself substantially contributes to a better stress response and your ability to cope with the slings and arrows of outrageous fortune. It's also good for you to be thinking about the welfare of others, which is a trait stressed in faith-based organizations and philosophies. I know this sounds naïve, but if everyone considered the impact of their actions on their fellow human beings, and practiced the 'Four Immeasurables' (see the Mind-Body chapter), this world would really be a much nicer place to live, and we'd all be less stressed and healthier.

Finally, Professor Brantner cautioned us to "not live alone". Although I took that to mean 'live in the same dwelling with someone else', now I believe he meant it was necessary to be interacting with others in meaningful ways. Engaging and contributing to the welfare of others is one of the most satisfying things that we as humans can do. It makes us feel good, it connects us to the web of life, and it saves us from the agony of too much self-preoccupation.

When I mentioned to my male friends that I was writing a book on health, each of them said, "Are you going to include a section on sex?" Most of my female friends, on the other hand, stressed 'relationships' as a cornerstone of health. Once again I may be drawing conclusions from too small a sample, but I think men consider sex to be necessary for a healthy life, while women tend to think of it as a bonus of a committed relationship. This certainly could just be a reflection of what kind of company I keep. At any rate, in alignment with the values of loving kindness, especially towards your partner, I would think that if one partner (no matter which) feels that sex is very important and healthful, then the other partner should make a loving attempt at it. Sex, like nutrition is a loaded subject.

In summary, you will become healthier and stay healthier if you live with a positive attitude, have a strong sense of self to overcome adversity and accomplish your goals, believe that there is more to life than just your own ego, and finally engage meaningfully with others through kindness. This kind of attitude will also enable you to incorporate the healthy habits outlined in this book into your life.

Chapter 7: Conclusion

"Be careful about reading health books. You may die of a misprint." - Mark Twain[37]

Overwhelmed? Don't be. It probably took you a long time to acquire some of your not-so-good habits. And hopefully not every area of your health needs work. Pick one area on which to concentrate your first efforts. All of the areas discussed work together in synergistic ways. For example, if you are exercising more, you will sleep better; and if you are sleeping better you will have more energy to exercise and you will be less hungry. As I said in the introduction, "Even if you choose to only adopt some of these suggestions, your general wellness can be improved with each area incorporated."

Just like starting an exercise program, start slow, don't overdo it or you will get discouraged and stop before your new behaviors become habits. The steps are 'easy' because you can take incremental baby steps to get you to your goals. Can't afford a white noise machine, yet your bedroom is noisy? Buy a simple set of ear plugs for sleeping and **use them,** or listen to a relaxing recording of your choice.

Take about 15 minutes a day (just before bedtime) to practice diaphragmatic breathing. You will start to learn better breathing as a habit while winding down to be more relaxed before falling asleep. At the same time you could also be listening to the relaxation recording with auto-suggestions included to reinforce these healthy behaviors. If you haven't already received your free relaxing download music, go to *http://www.radiance4u.com/*. All of the auto-suggestions on the recording are written out for you in the back of the checklist.

Can't remember all of the suggestions in this book? There is also a second free bonus download available for you. It is a PDF check-list summarizing the suggestions in this book. To download your free bonus checklist for you to follow, to help you to achieve your radiant health goals go to: *http://www.radiance4u.com/*

The rest is up to you. I hope that I have shown you the path to awesome radiant health. And if this book has helped you, **please contribute a positive review** of it for me where you purchased it. "Spread the health, and may radiant health be yours." Thank you, Jane Bersie

About the Author

Jane Bersie is a retired international computer consultant with over 40 years of experience, analyzing, designing, implementing and testing information technology systems for both small companies and Fortune 500 corporations. Her lifelong interest in maintaining optimum health was majorly influenced by the need to stay healthy and in top physical and mental condition to meet the demands of a high-stress computer consulting career. One has to be healthy in order to work long hours meeting critical deadlines while retaining the mental sharpness required to solve complex computer system issues.

In her lifelong quest to achieve and maintain optimal health, she has always belonged to a health club, exercised and danced regularly, read books, listened to audio programs and attended classes on every aspect of health she could find. Her learning experiences have included becoming a licensed esthetician and a licensed certified massage therapist through the Aveda Institute in Minneapolis. She is a certified aromatherapist, registered yoga instructor, semi-active Qigong practitioner, and registered Thai therapist. Additional training has included studying Thai healing techniques with multiple healing masters in Thailand, Thai acupressure, meditation, Spring Forest Qigong healing, DNA healing methods, Himalayan Institute Tantric yoga, nutrition, mantras, chakras, Ayurveda, beginning Reiki, and mind-body studies.

She has a Math degree from the University of Minnesota and a Master's degree in Education from St. Thomas University in St. Paul, Minnesota. She is currently retired, babysits for her wonderful grandchildren, and occasionally substitute teaches yoga classes.

[1] http://funnyfitnessquotes.tumblr.com/

[2] Jaslow, Ryan. *CDC: 80 percent of American adults don't get recommended exercise.* CBS NEWS May 3, 2013, 12:03 PM http://www.cbsnews.com/news/cdc-80-percent-of-american-adults-dont-get-recommended-exercise/

[3]"Physical Activity and Health – The Benefits of Physical Activity" *Centers for Disease Control and Prevention: Physical Activity for Everyone* USA.gov Feb. 11, 2011. http://www.cdc.gov/physicalactivity/everyone/health/index.html

[4] White, Betty. AARP Bulletin/Real Possibilities October, 2014

[5] "Why is Sleep Important?" *National Institute of Health: National Heart, Lung, and Blood Institute* USA.gov Feb 22, 2012 http://www.nhlbi.nih.gov/health/health-topics/topics/sdd/why.html

[6]"Why is Sleep Important?" *National Institute of Health: National Heart, Lung, and Blood Institute* USA.gov Feb 22, 2012 http://www.nhlbi.nih.gov/health/health-topics/topics/sdd/why.html

[7]Newsome, Melba; reviewed by Krucik, George, MD. "10 Natural Ways to Sleep Better" *Natural Sleeping Remedies* pg. 3 of 12, April 4, 2013 http://www.healthline.com/health-slideshow/natural-sleeping-remedies#3

[8] Paul, Marla. "Aerobic Exercise Relieves Insomnia – Boosting cardiovascular fitness improves sleep, vitality and mood for insomniacs" *Northwestern University News* Sept 15, 2010 http://www.northwestern.edu/newscenter/stories/2010/09/aerobic-exercise-relieves-insomnia.html

[9] Mercola, J. "Exposing Yourself to Light at Night Shuts Down Your Melatonin and Raises Your Cancer Risk" *The Many Health Benefits of Melatonin* March 19, 2013 http://articles.mercola.com/sites/articles/archive/2013/03/19/melatonin-benefits.aspx

[10] "Sleeping Tips & Tricks: National Sleep Foundation" *National Sleep Foundation* 2014 http://sleepfoundation.org/sleep-tools-tips/healthy-sleep-tips

[11] Mercola, J. "Exposing Yourself to Light at Night Shuts Down Your Melatonin and Raises Your Cancer Risk – Story at-a-glance" *The Many Health Benefits of Melatonin* March 19, 2013 http://articles.mercola.com/sites/articles/archive/2013/03/19/melatonin-benefits.aspx

[12]Newsome, Melba; reviewed by Krucik, George, MD. "10 Natural Ways to Sleep Better" Natural Sleeping Remedies pg. 8 of 12, April 4, 2013 http://www.healthline.com/health-slideshow/natural-sleeping-remedies#8

[13] Mayo Clinic. "Dog Tired? It Could Be Your Pooch" *ScienceDaily*, 15 February 2002 http://www.sciencedaily.com/releases/2002/02/020215070932.htm

[14] http://www.huffingtonpost.co.uk/2014/01/15/funny-quotes-diets-health-fitness_n_4601394.html

[15]*Food Dyes: A Rainbow of Risks* Center for Science in the Public Interest. 2014 http://www.cspinet.org/fooddyes/ Permission to quote dated 12/9/2014

[16] "Omega-3 Fatty Acids and Health - Fact Sheet for Health Professionals - Summary of key findings" U.S. Department of Health & Human Services: National Institutes of Health,

March, 2004 and February, 2005.
http://ods.od.nih.gov/factsheets/Omega3FattyAcidsandHealt
h-HealthProfessional/#h2

[17]Weil, Andrew M.D. "Q & A Library: Balancing Omega-3 and Omega-6?" DrWeil.com

http://www.drweil.com/drw/u/QAA400149/balancing-omega-
3-and-omega-6.html

[18] Martinez, Dr. Mario. *The Mind-Body Code: How the Mind Wounds and Heals the Body* (Audio book), Sounds True, 2009

[19] Robbins, Anthony (Tony). *Unlimited Power* (Audio Program), Nightingale Conant, 1986

[20] Lin, Master Chunyi. http://www.springforestqigong.com/

[21]Martinez, Dr. Mario. *The Mind-Body Code: How the Mind Wounds and Heals the Body* (Audio book), Sounds True, 2009

[22] Myss, Carolyn, Ph.D. *The Energetics of Healing*, DVD, Sounds True, 2004

[23] Martinez, Dr. Mario. *The Mind-Body Code: How the Mind Wounds and Heals the Body* (Audio book), Sounds True, 2009

[24] Sarno, John M.D. *Healing Back Pain: The Mind-Body Connection,* Grand Central Publishing, 2001

[25] Lin, Master Chunyi.
http://www.springforestqigong.com/index.php/master-
chunyi-lin

[26] Martinez, Dr. Mario. *Embodying the Four Immeasurables with Dr. Mario Martinez,* Jul 22, 2011

https://www.youtube.com/watch?v=A2Duu9JO6vg

[27] Chopra, Deepak. *The Seven Spiritual Laws of Success: A Practical Guide to the Fulfillment of Your Dreams*, New World Library/Amber-Allen Publishing, 1994

[28] Cousens, Gabriel M.D. *Conscious Eating*, North Atlantic Books, 2000

[29] Eveleth, Rose. "There are 37.2 Trillion Cells in Your Body" Smithsonian.com, October 2013 http://www.smithsonianmag.com/smart-news/there-are-372-trillion-cells-in-your-body-4941473/

[30]"International cyanide Management Code: Human Health Effects" extracted Sept 30, 2014 http://www.cyanidecode.org/cyanide-facts/environmental-health-effects

[31]Hendricks, Gay Ph.D. *Conscious Breathing – Breathwork for Health, Stress Release, and Personal Mastery*, Bantam Books, New York, 1995 p.4

[32] Rinpoche, Anyen; Choying Zangmo, Allison. *The Tibetan Yoga of Breath*, Shambala Publications, Boston, 2013 p.70

Lundberg, J.O. "Nitrous Oxide and the Paranasal Sinuses," *Anat Rec* 291 (2008): 1479-84, doi: 10.1002/ar.20782.

[33] Hendricks, Gay Ph.D. *Conscious Breathing – Breathwork for Health, Stress Release, and Personal Mastery*, Bantam Books, New York, 1995 p.5

[34] Hendricks, Gay Ph.D. *Conscious Breathing – Breathwork for Health, Stress Release, and Personal Mastery*, Bantam Books, New York, 1995 p.4

[35]

http://quotations.about.com/od/funnyquotesbyauthor/a/Charli

e-Chaplin-Quotes.htm extracted 12/13/2014

[36] "Positive Thinking: Stop negative thoughts to reduce stress - The health benefits of positive thinking", *Healthy Lifestyle – Stress Management*, Mayo Clinic, referenced 12/11/2014
http://www.mayoclinic.org/healthy-living/stress-management/in-depth/positive-thinking/art-20043950

[37] "Major Attitude",
http://www.seniorresource.com/attitude.htm extracted 12/11/2014

Made in the USA
Middletown, DE
27 December 2024

68298358R00031